WHY YOU CAN'T FOCUS

How to regain your attention and live an ordered life in an unordered society

JOHN STROUT

TABLE OF CONTENTS

HELP YOUR HEALTH BY CHANGING YOUR DIET

Sugar should be reduced or eliminated.

Caffeine should be used with caution.

Stay Hydrated by Breathing Deeply

TAKE TIME TO BE IN NATURE

RULE 20-8-2

REGULAR EXERCISE

CONCLUSION

INTRODUCTION

Life becomes a problem when you can't concentrate. Everything you do is more difficult and time consuming than it should be. When your attention wanders, it affects your work, school, relationships, and confidence.

It's infuriating to spend more time accomplishing less!

Focus, on the other hand, is not an innate attribute or talent. It's a talent that can be honed.

Every day, you rely on concentration to go through job or school. You won't be able to think properly, focus on a task, or sustain your attention if you can't concentrate.

You may also notice that you are unable to think clearly, which may have an impact on your decision-making. A difficulty to concentrate can be caused by or contributed to by a variety of medical issues.

Your mind wanders or you start scrolling through your phone every time you sit down to work. Does this ring a bell? Most people have problems concentrating at times. However, if this happens frequently, you may question why you can't stay focused.

Many factors, such as daily behaviors, might impair your capacity to concentrate, and in some situations, a health problem may be to blame.

WHY ARE YOU UNABLE TO FOCUS?

MULTITASKING

It may appear like working on a report while answering emails and listening to a conference call is a good way to save time. However, juggling too many things at once might backfire. Our brains are designed to focus on one task at a time. According to research, switching gears all the time makes you less productive and more likely to make mistakes.

And doing one thing at a time is the only way to genuinely pay attention.

The goal of multitasking – to get more done in less time is already detrimental. It's common knowledge that you can only think about one thing at a time.

When you multitask, your brain must quickly switch from one task to the next. This can squander up to 40% of your working time.

STRESS

When you're stressed, experts believe the survival center of your brain takes over. The areas of your brain that control attention and reasoning, for example, do not receive as much energy.

You may have noticed that short-term stress, such as working under a deadline, enhances focus for a brief period of time. However, this rate cannot be maintained.

Stress affects your brain's health and function over time, resulting in a shorter attention span, poor memory, and poor judgment.

Chronic stress has a subtle effect on your brain. It really accelerates the aging of your brain by causing it to lose enough brain cells to shrink.

SLEEP DEPRIVATION

When you're fatigued, it's difficult to pay attention. This is because while you sleep, your brain cells regenerate and recover. When you don't get enough sleep, they don't work as well. According to studies, missing even one night of sleep makes it difficult to concentrate and shut out distractions. Sleep deprivation impairs the ability of brain cells to communicate with one another.

As a result, focus, memory, mood, and overall mental function suffer. Sleep deprivation has the same effect on your mental performance as being intoxicated!

Apart from dreaming, a lot happens in your brain while you sleep.

Your brain is busily generating new brain cells, integrating memories from the day, and cleaning, mending, and reorganizing itself while you sleep.

CONSUMPTION OF HIGH-SUGAR OR HIGH-FAT FOODS.

Sugar generates a spike in blood sugar followed by a drop in energy. In the meanwhile, diets high in harmful saturated fat may cause inflammation in the brain. Women performed worse on an attention test after eating a dinner heavy in unsaturated fat, according to one study.

YOUR BRAIN DOESN'T GET ENOUGH FUEL.

Your brain is a high-performance organ that requires a lot of energy, oxygen, water, and nutrients to function properly. It's more difficult to concentrate when your blood sugar drops.

What you eat has a big impact on how well your brain performs all of its activities, including focusing.

CONDITIONS OF HEALTH

Finally, there are a variety of underlying medical and mental health issues that can affect brain function and focus.

Anxiety, depression, schizophrenia, post-traumatic stress disorder, dementia, and, of course, attention issues may all wreak havoc on your capacity to concentrate.

The following medical conditions have been linked to a loss of focus:

- A case of altitude sickness
- Poisoning by carbon monoxide

- Diabetes

- Damage to the head

- Illness of the heart

- Heatstroke

- Hypothermia

- Infections

- Illness of the lung

- Malnutrition

- Abuse of substances

- Thyroid problems

What are the signs and symptoms of inability to FOCUS?

People react differently to being unable to concentrate. You may experience the following symptoms:

- Being unable to recall events from a brief period of time
- Sitting for long periods of time
- Having trouble thinking clearly
- Frequently misplacing items or having trouble remembering where they are.
- Being unable to make decisions
- Inability to complete difficult jobs
- Unable to concentrate due to a lack of physical or mental energy
- Committing thoughtless errors

You may realize that concentrating is more difficult at certain times of the day or in specific environments.

Others may observe that you look to be preoccupied. Due to a lack of focus, you may miss appointments or meetings.

Techniques for enhancing Regaining your focus

TIME BLOCK

Do you have a lot on your plate right now? Set aside time for each work, such as a half-hour each morning and afternoon to check email or return phone calls. This eliminates the need to switch back and forth between tasks.

REDUCE THE NUMBER OF DISTRACTIONS.

When you need to concentrate, try to find a peaceful place. Remove everything that is constantly vying for your attention. For a while, you might wish to turn off the television or radio and turn off your phone notifications.

POMODORO TECHNIQUE

It is a time management strategy.

To begin, make a clear statement about what you want to achieve.

After that, get rid of any evident distractions that are under your power.

Then, for the next 25 minutes, set a timer for 25 minutes and give the task at hand your entire concentration to the best of your ability.

Don't berate yourself if your mind wanders; merely bring it back to your short-term aim.

Take a break when the timer goes off, then repeat as needed.

You're teaching your brain to become better at paying attention by simply focusing on one subject during these 25-minute intervals.

MEDITATION

Meditation is one of the most effective ways to enhance focus and reduce stress.

Meditation promotes the alpha brainwave state, which improves focus and concentration, stimulates creativity, and causes deep relaxation.

It has firmly established itself as a popular discipline.

Meditation has been tested by the US Marine Corps, and it has been found to assist soldiers stay focused and calm under duress.

Employees at major corporations are encouraged to meditate. Employees who meditate are happier, healthier, and less likely to ruminate or be distracted, according to these firms.

DOPAMINE LEVELS INCREMENT

Food, vitamins, and physical activity are all natural ways to boost dopamine levels.

Appropriate goal planning, on the other hand, is one way to increase dopamine while also ensuring that you get more done.

If you follow sports, you've probably seen athletes perform a victory dance or raise their fists in victory. Their euphoria is caused by a surge of dopamine.

You can execute your own "victory dance" whenever you achieve a goal.

By reducing major goals into many smaller goals, you can trick your brain into producing more of this "motivation molecule."

You'll experience a small rush of dopamine after each action is completed. Each surge of dopamine aids you in remaining concentrated and motivated.

THE RULE OF 'FIVE MORE'

This is a basic technique for improving concentration. When you feel like quitting, just do five more – five more minutes, five more exercises, five more pages – and your attention will be extended. The rule pushes you just past the point of frustration while also aiding in the development of mental attention. It's both a sort of training and a method of accomplishing something.

It would appear that sitting motionless is a simple task. However, it is more difficult than it appears. It's similar to meditation, which can help you concentrate better. In this scenario, though, simply sit in a comfortable, supported position for five minutes and do nothing. It can be used as a break between tasks. If you already meditate, you can combine this with breathing for a quick "time out."

COUNTING BACKWARDS

Counting backwards is another great method for improving concentration. Counting backwards in sevens from 1,000 may appear to be an exasperating activity, but it does need intense concentration: try it.

It necessitates perseverance and the use of various skills, which for some may entail visualizing the numbers while counting. Whatever it takes, remain at it long enough to completely focus, and you'll discover that you've temporarily freed your mind of everything else.

Similarly, spelling words backwards is a wonderful technique to focus on: start with simple words like dog, box, and cup, then work your way up to longer terms like cushion, blonde, effort, and number, gradually increasing the length and complexity of the word. This is an activity that can be expanded upon.

WATCHING THE CLOCK

For this, you'll need an old-fashioned clock face with hands and a second hand. Begin with the second hand at 12 o'clock and concentrate solely on its movement around the clock face, allowing no other ideas to enter your mind. Wait until the second hand is at the 12 again before starting again if your concentration is broken by a stray thought. It's more difficult than it appears, and it might be annoying at first, but once you've mastered it, you'll find it easy to use whenever you need to focus your thoughts.

POWER NAP

When you don't receive the necessary 7 to 9 hours of sleep every night, a nap can help fill the void.

Afternoon power naps of 20 minutes can help you stay focused, awake, and productive for the rest of the day.

It has been discovered that napping increases productivity and lasts longer than caffeine consumption.

HELP YOUR HEALTH BY CHANGING YOUR DIET

Your diet should resemble the Mediterranean "real food" diet rather than the normal American "processed food" diet for best attention.

Here are a few dietary tips that can help you focus more effectively.

Sugar should be reduced or eliminated.

Dietary advice has become unnecessarily convoluted and contentious, but scientists agree on one thing: sugar is terrible for your mental and physical health.

Sugar has a bad impact on your memory, emotions, and attention span. It alters the patterns of your brainwaves, making it difficult to think coherently.

Sugar causes inflammation in the brain, which has been related to poor focus and a variety of mental health issues.

Sugar causes your blood sugar to go up and down like a roller coaster. Low blood sugar will undoubtedly cause you to lose attention.

Caffeine should be used with caution.

Caffeine is widely used for its ability to improve focus, alertness, memory, and productivity, although it is not appropriate in all circumstances.

If you use caffeine, you must be careful about how much you take. More than you're used to can make you nervous, and too little can leave you with your head buried in your desk – neither extreme will help you concentrate.

Caffeine can make stress worse and make anxiety symptoms worse.

It lowers blood flow to the brain, which is bad for brain health and function, as you might expect.

Blood flow to the brain provides oxygen and nutrients that your brain cells require; poor focus and concentration are indicators of decreased blood flow to the brain.

Caffeine should be consumed in moderation and in nearly the same amount every day if you use it.

Caffeine should be treated as the psychoactive drug that it is, and used with caution.

Stay Hydrated by Breathing Deeply

Water and oxygen are two elements that are often forgotten but are essential necessary for proper brain function.

Your brain is made up of 73 percent water, and even a small amount of dehydration can have a significant influence on your capacity to concentrate.

TAKE TIME TO BE IN NATURE

Spending time in nature helps to cleanse your thoughts and restore your ability to concentrate.

Viewing nature landscapes helps to regulate the autonomic nervous system's activity, resulting in a state of relaxation.

Spending an hour connecting with nature can boost your attention span and memory by 20%. There are some simple workarounds if spending time in nature every day isn't possible.

- Take a moment to look out a window.
- Looking at a green roof for just 40 seconds increased concentration and focus, according to one research.

- If you don't have a view, place houseplants in your home or office, keep nature images on your desk, or set a wallpaper of natural wonders or landscapes on your computer monitor if you don't have one.

RULE 20-8-2

The average American spends ten hours every day sitting. We're getting big, exhausted, and ill from all of our sitting. It's also robbing us of our capacity to concentrate.

You could use a standing desk or a sit-stand workstation, but this isn't always feasible.

Alternatively, you can use the 20-8-2 rule.

Sit for a maximum of 20 minutes every half-hour, stand for 8, and move about for 2.

REGULAR EXERCISE

Regular physical activity improves your ability to focus, learn, and recall.

It can assist you in de-stressing, sleeping better, and reducing stress. It also helps to reduce inflammation and promotes the formation of new brain cells. In the long run, this may help you think more clearly.

According to a famous specialist, exercise can help the mind focus just as well as attention deficit medicines.

It is not necessary to engage in strenuous exercise to reap the benefits.

Walking is not only one of the best all-around exercises, but it also helps you clear your mind and think more clearly.

When it comes to physical activity, how much is enough?

According to new research, the minimal amount of time you need to keep cognitively sharp is 8 hours every month.

CONCLUSION

These tactical adjustments won't be enough to wean your system on their own, but they'll go a long way toward making it easier for you to do so.

Still, keep in mind that altering your brain's most often used neural pathways takes time and demands a lot of discipline at initially.

So, once you've set these things up, concentrate on the positive habits we discussed before, such as time blocking and regular exercise.

That ability to concentrate intently will eventually return.